My Dear Cancer Cells ...

An Intimate Talk about Unruly Cells in Your Body and How to Take Control

Jimmy Diaz, MD

ISBN 979-8-89485-375-8 (Paperback)
ISBN 979-8-89485-376-5 (Digital)

Covenant Books
11661 Hwy 707
Murrells Inlet, SC 29576
www.covenantbooks.com

Contents

Prologue

I am a physician, first trained in internal medicine and fifteen years later in alternative medicine. At the beginning of my private practice, I was discovering cancer about once every three to six months. Now I discover fully developed tumors at least once a week. That is unacceptable given the level of technological development of our society, but still, it happens. For over fifteen years, the method discussed here has helped hundreds of patients. You are next.

There are two trends in the approach to cancer.

One, the mainstream medical establishment's way of "let's kill everything."

And two, the regenerative medicine approach of "Let's figure out what is happening, then let's turn that reaction off, so cancer does not come back, and then kill or control the mutated cells, while the good, healthy ones are left intact to repair and thrive."

Which one do you think is better for you?

Each person is different, and the cause of the disease is also different in each person. This book is intended to guide your thoughts about the condition called cancer so that you can collect your feelings, lose your fears, and move on to a solid plan to go back to health.

Don't let past results distort the way you think about your future. Let the past stay where it belongs: in the past. Your future has not been written yet, but it is been decided with each step that you take today. I hope that you come to realize that there is only one of you and that you are special. Body and soul must work together to win this one. In the end, it is the journey that defines us.

So sit back and learn. This is a completely different approach. I purposely wrote a very small book so that you can read it without getting tired. In many of you, chemotherapy and radiotherapy have already zapped the energy out of your life. I also try not to bother you with technical and scientific terms. This small book is written in simple English, hoping to address a big problem, fast, so you can start this one journey, fighting a lethal disease as soon as possible.

That smile, when you finally realize that you can do this, is the end of the condition that they call cancer and the beginning of the condition that I call HEALTH!

Well, let's start learning so that you can get back to happiness. I will take you by the hand. You will never be alone.

Chapter 1

Experiencing Cancer, Not Suffering from It

Everything happens in phases; cancer is not the exception. It starts as an inflammation that, if not resolved, produces genetic changes, with the final phase being a tumor. A tumor is nothing else than a bunch of similar cells grouped together. Each stage produces different symptoms and thus needs different treatment protocols. But the main thing is to remain positive and concentrate on beating this thing. The tumor is the last phase in the development of cancer. It means that the cancer has matured.

As emotions are vital influences in health and illness, that is the first point that needs to be visited. You can do a self-examination of your mental health status, but sometimes, we may benefit from a counselor or psychologist.

It is vital that you be at peace with yourself. Yes, you must forgive others for what they may have done to you, but you must also forgive yourself.

Guilty feelings just feed the development of cancer because it decreases the immune system's ability to recognize and kill mutated cells. Lift yourself up. Smile, not just at others, but at you.

The body functions as a whole. Every cell has unique functions that, together, as a tissue, influence other tissues, organs, and systems. For example, serotonin produced in the intestines is used by the brain. When thyroid function is low, the serotonin production in the gut is reduced. When the brain does not have enough of it, it gets into a depressed state, and you feel sad. See, problems in one area result in symptoms in another seemingly unrelated organ.

The process also works in reverse. Anxiety or sadness for prolonged periods end up affecting organ function. Yes, unchecked emotions make you sick.

Now do you see why we must resolve emotions? Many patients who are declared cancer-free by their oncologist actually are just tumor-free. There is a recurrence in a few months or years, but it is not because the cancer came back; it is because it never left. But don't worry. That is why you are reading this book so that you can learn how to totally remove it from your body, and knowledge is power.

If you were already diagnosed with cancer, after the initial shock, lift your head and say with confidence: "Cancer, you are not going to beat me, so start packing because soon you will be history." And you will say that with confidence, knowing in your heart that it will be so.

The most powerful treatment against cancer is you. You will win this one.

You will have to make changes in your life if you want to beat this thing. You need to get in the mindset that you have to do what you have to do to save your life. Staying idle and waiting for death is NOT an option and is not fair to you, your loved ones, and the people who depend on you. Attitude, diet, sleep, hydration, supplements, daily activities; all these things must be examined, evaluated, and improved.

No problem. Your goal is to survive. Each person has a different challenge. So each one of us will come out of this a bit different. But it is your willingness to live that will give you the edge, the chance to make it. I keep emphasizing this because your attitude is the most important part of your recovery. Separate yourself from the grief of having this diagnosis and move on to the recovery phase. You will make it.

Even with cancer in your body, you can have a happy, prosperous, and fruitful existence. Before you were diagnosed and before symptoms were very evident, cancer was in you. Probably, it took four or five years for cancer to develop into the present stage. It was developing in silence for a long time. And you were doing well, feeling good, enjoying life.

Every day, you went to work, did your daily activities, visited your relatives, enjoyed your family, etc., etc. Things got worse after the diagnosis. So let's get back to a stable, calm state not just in your mind but also in your body.

You are one organism. Head to toe, you are still just one being. So let's now study you as a whole.

Assignment: Think of a happy moment before you were told of

your diagnosis. Smile and relieve that moment. Talk to someone who was involved in that happy memory. Immerse yourself completely in the experience. Stay there. Take a deep breath. Now say to yourself: I will be that happy again for a long time!

Thanks be to the Lord!

Chapter 2

You as a Whole

Most people go through life without analyzing themselves, without truly knowing not just *who* but *what* they are.

Yes, you have a name, you are male or female, you have a job with a job description, and you have a position in your family (parent, child, sibling, spouse), but you are a lot more physically.

Physiologically speaking, we are a collection of elements put together in organic form. Iron, calcium, potassium, and oxygen—they all exist in vast quantities in the soil and the environment. But something called life is what makes those elements work together. Everything we are made of is present in the soil and in the air. But by themselves, those elements do not work. It is not until they are incorporated as cells and then tissues that the thing starts to function and make sense.

A heart valve by itself is nothing. When it becomes part of the heart, then it becomes functional. A heart by itself cannot do anything. It needs blood, arteries, veins, and capillaries to be called a circulatory system. The circulatory system needs a place to pump blood. As you see, everything is connected. Every organ is part of, and depends on, everything else. But without guidance, we would be vegetables, just existing. Thus, the mind.

And the mind is not the same thing as the brain.

The mind: self-awareness is what makes you unique and special. Consciousness is what relates us to the environment and each other. That is how you experience joy and sadness, love and hunger, creativity and sexual desire.

Then comes the soul. More difficult to explain, yes, but not any less vital. There reside moral issues like celibacy, faithfulness, and suicide. Those things that are not shared with the rest of the living creatures of this one planet.

All that is you. Precious and unique. Today, of a certain age. Different in all aspects from everyone else but also changing every day.

Every breath you take changes you because it may have more or less oxygen, humidity, pollen, contaminants, perfumes, etc. Every bite of food changes you for the better or for the worse. Nutrients, artificial colorings, preservatives, hydration, and free radicals all come in through your mouth and the digestive system and is all your choice, for the most part.

You are also a son or daughter, a brother or sister, a husband or wife, a mom, or an aunt or uncle, a cousin—a family unit. Even if you live alone, there is a bunch out there genetically related to you. Then come friends and those related by marriage, coworkers, and the thousands that you interact with but will never get to know. Nobody is isolated. We influence each other.

Everything that you experience results in a response from your body:

an emotion. Thunder results in fear. The first snow of the season gets you in a good mood. Those emotions also affect your health. They may be positive, or they may be negative but affected you will be.

Now is the time to ask yourself: What is my condition today according to MY own reality?

Assignment: (Pencil your answer to the right.)

Do I eat well?

Do I rest enough?

Do I consider myself a happy person?

What is my health status?

Why am I sick?

Only you can answer that.

Now let's move on. We need a plan of action. No war was ever won without a definite plan. First, we will find out where you are. The approach to get you back on the road to recovery is based on where you are now.

———

Chapter 3

First Stop the Growth

Can you put out a fire that is being fed by gasoline? Of course not. We must first turn that gas valve off. Then we have a chance to successfully put out the flames. Same with any type of disease or illness.

Information is key. You need a *physical exam*. Someone needs to put eyes on you, your hair, your eyes, your tongue, your skin. Your appearance says a ton about you as a living organism. As physicians, many have lost the art of examination. Family physicians and alternative medicine physicians are still the best at this. Schedule a good, thorough exam.

Then tests are needed to scientifically confirm what the physical exam suggests. *Laboratory testing* should include CBC to examine the number and size of red cells, white cells, platelets, and a complete metabolic profile to check liver and kidney function, electrolytes, and glucose. Other particularly important tests are a full thyroid panel, vitamin D3, growth hormone, reproductive hormones, early morning cortisol, urine analysis and stool analysis, the presence of fungus in your system, food sensitivities, and inflammation levels.

More advanced testing may include cancer markers, endoscopies, low-dose radiological exams, thermal imaging, and quantum magnetic resonance imaging. That is how we diagnose in our office.

My evaluation of patients includes these tests. I get lots of information without being too invasive or too expensive.

Although most patients come to us already with the results of many tests, seldom have their previous physicians checked their hormones or tested for systemic candidiasis, growth hormone, or vitamin D levels.

The food that you eat, and water and other drinks could be making you sick and working against your healing. Don't wait. Clean up your diet.

It is important to have a balanced diet. Carbs are especially important for energy. Without energy, there is nothing that your cells can do to get rid of the very big, strong, and powerful cancer cells.

Protein is very important. Animal protein has essential amino acids that your body needs to build human proteins. But hormones and fat are to be watched for. Lean cuts of hormone-free animals are what you need to look for. Also, protein needs in your diet are moderate. Your body produces human proteins. All you need is to eat the basic molecules.

I argue against biopsies unless it is during surgery and is excisional, meaning that the whole tumor is removed for examination. A tumor is a closed entity surrounded by alpha-fetoprotein and a crust of protein and collagen. It grows from the inside. When a biopsy is taken, the seal is broken, and cancer cells leak out of the tumor and escape. That may explain why we found metastasis months after biopsy when there were none at the time.

When a woman is pregnant, the baby is a foreign body to her immune system. The immune system of the mother should attack that baby. It does not because the immune system is programmed not to attack alpha-fetoprotein. The baby is covered by that protein.

Cancer tumors also surround themselves with this substance to be invisible to the immune system. The only way that it is normal to have any levels of this substance is if you are pregnant. Positive levels in a man or a woman who is not pregnant indicate cancer until proven otherwise. High doses of vitamin C wash away alpha-fetoprotein so that your immune system can see your tumor and destroy it.

Bring all those tests and reports to the evaluation appointment. Otherwise, our health-care providers can order the tests that we feel necessary. In our office, we see very few patients a day so that we can spend as much time as each one needs. Hopefully, your physician will do the same.

Once we know your actual health status, the next step is to check your *emotional balance*. We are not talking necessarily about psychologists, but a counselor should be invited to help you analyze any present or past source of emotional stress. Half the battle is just to identify. Sometimes, just talking about it is enough relief to turn that bad experience off. Why is this so important? Emotions are related to certain types of diseases, and symptoms may manifest themselves in a specific area or system. I am not a psychologist, so the conversation here will be short.

For more information about this, please look into the work of Dr. Hamer, the German doctor who discovered these relationships between emotions and disease and studied them in a scientific way. His book *Summary of the New Medicine* is in English. Also check out www.newmedicine.ca. Other cultures have known this for centuries.

Now the big one: *food intake.*

It will help you to write everything that you eat for at least three or four days (food log). The idea is to analyze your diet for quantity, quality, type of nutrients, both present and lacking, toxins, timing of intake, etc. The content of your diet may be a very important clue on what is going on here.

When your organism processes what you eat (note that I didn't say food because not everything we put in our mouths has nutritional value), there are some particles left over by that process. These are called free radicals. These are small molecules, generally electrically charged, that will attach themselves to important areas of the cell wall and suppress its function.

Heavy metals are a significant cause of disease. If not removed, they may lead to high blood pressure, high blood sugar, and even Alzheimer's disease. Many grew up with lead paint in their homes and cribs, leaded gasoline, or worked in contaminated environments. Amalgams, aluminum cookware and cans, and even antiperspirants and antiacids transfer heavy metals to us. The only test that I recommend for heavy metal toxicity is a provocative test. This test consists of an IV that contains calcium EDTA, a substance that makes heavy metals electrically neutral and excretable so that they can be measured in your urine and feces. Blood is not a reliable way to test for heavy metals because there is not a binding protein that will keep metals in your blood and create a steady state. For example, by the time lead shows in your blood in any significant level you are already poisoned. We hope to find it at still only mildly toxic levels when there is still a chance to help you. Many other heavy metals can cause disease, like mercury, cadmium, gadolinium, and arsenic. They all need to be removed by chelation, a series of IV treatments, based on calcium EDTA and other substances that bind to heavy metals and free radicals.

Medical imaging contrast also could be a source of toxins like gadolinium.

Plastics are artificially formed molecules, and the body does not know what to do with them, so they are parked in tissues and eventually interfere with that particular tissue's function.

There should not be a "safe" level of these toxins in humans. Any amount present should be cause for alarm. Chelation should be started immediately.

The *immune system* is a critical component of this plan. A weak immune system is not the cause of cancer but has allowed it to grow unimpeded.

Not acceptable, Soldier! Our immune system does three things: maintenance, repair, and vigilance. It needs to be optimized so that we can have a happy outcome.

Maintenance. Every day, during our activities of daily living, we have normal wear and tear of our cells and tissues. For example, when we eat, the stomach produces acid, which is used to destroy the layers of the food that we ingest in order to get the nutrients. A good side effect is that most bacteria in your food can't survive in this low pH (acid) environment. But the bad side of this is that the acid also deteriorates the lining of the stomach. As we sleep, the body repairs that lining.

The body is very busy at night, as you can see. The lining of the stomach is replaced daily.

Repair. When we have injuries, for example, a torn ligament, the function changes from maintenance to repair. It is a more intense function and a different work altogether, the difference between replacing a worn tire vs repairing a hole from a nail. Growth hormone and stem cells do their best job during this function.

Vigilance. This function is to keep intruders away, fighting bacteria, viruses, fungi, etc. Cancer is also an intruder. Cancer cells are genetically different and must be removed. This is also the role of your immune system. But to destroy the cancer cells, the body needs to identify them as bad actors. T Cells do the detective work here, identifying cells that have mutated into bad cells. These cells are marked for destruction, then the macrophages, or really big white cells, move in and engulf the cells previously marked by the T cells. Only cells marked are removed; thus, the importance of the T cells function.

The immune system is very important and has various functions. It is as if the same person did custodian work, changed light bulbs, repaired anything broken, and also became the security guard. Amazing!

The intestines produce most of the substances used by your immune system. They also produce most of the substances used by your brain. Poor gut function leads to deficiencies in production and deficiency in absorption of the substances needed for the tissues to repair and produce hormones and enzymes. But the gut also helps to get rid of unwanted stuff that piggy backs in our food and also helps eliminate waste from our cells.

Leaky gut is a term to describe a condition in which a sick intestinal membrane allows unwanted and sometimes dangerous substances to be absorbed into the bloodstream—

incredible system. But nobody cares about gut health. We do!

Eat minimally processed, fresh foods. Take probiotics to reseed your intestines of good bacteria.

Well, now that you know what it does and how important it is, it should come front and center in your fight against cancer. Choose what you put in your mouth carefully. Health and disease depend on it.

Assignment

Name two artificial food colorants.

Name the substance in soda that pulls calcium from your bones and makes your blood acid.

Make a list of everything that you ate today that was not 100 percent natural.

Chapter 4

Now Let's Move
In for the Kill

As we said before, imagine a fire fed by gasoline. It would be futile to try to extinguish it if gasoline keeps pouring in. So first, you turn off the gasoline valve, then you can extinguish the fire. Same with cancer. We must turn off the cause; if not, we will never get rid of the malignant bastard.

Now let us be honest: I believe in the removal of any tumor, completely, if possible. Metastasis (tumors in other areas of your body) comes from already established tumors. So the moment a tumor is discovered, the first step is to take it out immediately, if that is feasible. I do not care if it is Friday afternoon or Christmas Eve. The moment a tumor is discovered, we need to separate it from you ASAP if removal does not pose any danger to your life. Don't wait!

Cancer stages are numbered after the metastasis:

0 = no metastasis to
4 = many tumors away from the
main area involved

Talk to a competent surgeon. The tumor needs to be removed without biopsy, taken out whole, and then sent to pathology. Don't let them open you, take a biopsy of the tumor, wait for the preliminary report, and then proceed with removal. That is, in many cases, a death sentence because tumor cells will leak out and produce metastasis (distant tumors).

If the tumor is not at a place that is easy to remove, then leave it alone. Start other means of treatment immediately.

I have not seen a tumor that does not respond to high doses of vitamin C.

Agree with your doctor about a good plan to do this. It is reasonably cheap and simple and will not interfere with chemo or radiation.

High-dose vitamin C treatment

I recommend that you start with an IV vitamin C infusion of twenty-five thousand milligrams. Then increase to fifty thousand milligrams and move on to seventy-five thousand milligrams and one hundred thousand milligrams as you can tolerate.

Hydrogen peroxide is a great tool for its antimalignancy and antibiotic properties.

Depending on the patient's condition when they first get to our office, we may provide infusions from twice a week for the very ill to every other week for those not as affected.

The spleen needs to remove the carcasses of those cells and bacteria and viruses that are killed. We need to give that organ time to keep up. Millions of cancer cells will die with each treatment. Your spleen will be busy. If overwhelmed, the patient will feel really tired, and blood cells will suffer the effects of the spleen's function being backed up.

Patients in remission receive an infusion of vitamin C every 10 to 12 weeks as we remain vigilant to make sure that the malignant process does not come back.

A protocol with high-quality oral supplements and medication (if warranted) will be implemented from day one. The goal is to provide support to your body as it strains to get rid of the malignancy. Not only the sick tissues will need attention, but the other organs will also feel the load of this effort. They must be monitored and supported too.

Vitamin D is a great cancer fighter. I recommend ten thousand international units by mouth daily to keep blood levels at 80–100 ng/ml. Do not take a weekly dose. Your body will metabolize it in three to four days, and then the rest of the week, you will not be protected.

I have seen many patients die of the side effects of chemo or radiation. The cure was worse than the disease. A good regenerative medicine clinic pays attention to ALL of you to keep you safe.

Laboratory testing and proper imaging may be needed to see how you are responding to the treatment. The plan is active and fluid. Your treatment may be modified as we go, according to the feedback from your symptoms and testing.

Recent advances in cancer treatment have been made in the field of immunotherapy. As we discover ways that the body uses to attack a tumor, new substances are made to enhance the attacks by your immune system. The research is promising. But there is still much to learn about side effects, both short and long-term.

Emotions. This is very important for the present and future of your condition. Check emotional stress and deal with it. If you don't do this, the problem will likely resurface again. A stressful job, a toxic personal relationship, children or elders in significant need of care, poor living conditions, guilty feelings—you get the idea.

Diet. Processed sugar is definitely unhealthy if heavily processed and in large quantities. I suggest following a diabetic diet but without artificial sweeteners. Cancer needs lots of energy; thus, the weight loss of people affected by this condition. Stop feeding it. Actually, let's starve the thing. Sugar also helps fungi to grow, which could mediate genetic mutation.

Limit anything artificial and with preservatives. Food coloring and artificial flavors are not good for anybody but very bad for people with mutating cells. Artificial mint flavor has recently been associated with cancer. Red ink in tattoos also has been associated with skin tumors. Fluoride is not what we were led to believe. Eat as naturally as possible. Choose organic, but confirm the source. Not everything that says organic actually is.

No GMOs (genetically modified organisms), please! We depend on naturally grown food to be digested as intended. GMOs are different from the original in many ways. Genetically speaking, they are a variant of the natural organism. Our body will incorporate that altered genetic stuff into our cells. Not good at all!

Antioxidants. This means the opposite of oxidants. If a piece of metal is rusty, it has been oxidized. Damaged by oxygen. Yes, the same oxygen so needed for life can also cause damage if not handled properly. It is because it is electrically charged. Other substances are also electrically charged and are a result of our metabolism. They are at the end of molecules that we need and eat, and when metabolized, the body removes and discards that part. Antioxidants attach themselves to those molecules, making a neutrally charged complex that is easily removed from the body by mostly the liver, spleen, and kidneys. We need plenty of antioxidants on our plate every day.

Anything that turns dark when exposed to oxygen has antioxidants. For example, apples, bananas, cabbage, etc. Eat more of this stuff. You will also find them as supplements. To date, the best antioxidant is coffee. The health benefits of wine come from the antioxidant properties of red grapes.

Direct cell death. We don't have time to waste. The growth of a tumor must be stopped at once. Start with IV vitamin C as soon as possible. It will kill mutating cells, regardless of the origin. Tumors will start to reduce in size as you use high-dose vitamin C. All cancer tumors are susceptible to vitamin C. Until you can get to a physician who can administer vitamin C intravenously, start taking six thousand milligrams to nine thousand milligrams a day by mouth in three divided doses. In severe cases, I also include IV hydrogen peroxide along with some of the IV vitamin C treatments with caution because it can affect your veins. Do not take oral peroxide.

Mold and fungus. Genes must mutate for a normal cell to become cancerous—one of the theories of how this happens points to fungus. Fungal chemistry may allow for wrong gene splitting. With defective genes, mutations take place.

High sugar intake promotes fungus overgrowth in the body. Early humans' diet was mostly fruits and other herbs. No complex or modified carbs. No high fructose corn syrup. Diabetes probably was not among our ancestors.

Check your home and place of work for mold. Clean or leave immediately if mold is present.

I like to include an antifungal in my cancer treatment protocol to prevent new cells from mutating.

Chapter 5

Be at Peace with Yourself, Be Positive

Stop thinking of past experiences. You are here and now. Let's just think about changing course. A map is only good if you know (a) where you are and (b) where you want to go.

Your health map today looks like this:

Point A: You are sick.
Point B: You want to be healthy again.

Good. Now that we have a road map, we can start our trip from point A to point B. Let's find health in your life map.

It is very important for you to be positive, to think that you will be okay. Think of the day when you will receive the news that your cancer is gone! Smiles, hugs, tears of joy then to celebrate.

Once you are done with active treatment, plan something fun, a vacation, visit friends and family—have a party! Start planning now. This is your reward for winning this fight!

Think: "I AM CANCER-FREE!" Create positive thoughts. You see, everything was a thought before it was created. Somebody imagined my desk before it was built. The same with my pen. Someone imagined it, made drawings, and then it was created. So see yourself free of cancer, then act like there is nothing wrong with you.

Express that you are cancer-free even before you actually are. Make it a fact in your mind. Smile. Now that you know that you will be fine, let others know as well. Get rid of those pajamas, get dressed, go out. Get your hair done and your nails. Buy new clothes. Go to a concert, to a fair. Visit your favorite restaurant. Guys, go do something fun, buy new tools, spend a couple of hours at a car show, go to the movies. It is *your* new future, so do something that you like.

Get rid of that sick, losing attitude typical of an oncologist's office. This thing is on its way out of your body and your life. Let's celebrate!

Be thankful. Appreciate every day that you have. Don't waste it. Balance your day: rest-fun-work-sleep. Bring something with you to share when you visit someone. Share food and a card. Any gift is good. Share, share, share!

Talk. Share your emotions. Talk about the good old days, about good times. Find your old pictures, play your preferred songs, relive old trips, go to a family reunion or plan one. Feel good about your future, and do away with negatives in your past. Today is the beginning of your new life. Every day, it starts all over again.

Just fill your days with happiness.

Next, find a physician that believes in life, that believes in you. Don't stop your oncology treatments, but add a reasonable alternative medicine plan. Supplement with your regenerative medicine doctor's advice.

Vitamin C, vitamin D, hydrogen peroxide, peptides, stem cells, and other treatments have proven for decades that they work. No reason they will not help you. Every little bit helps.

Newer oncology treatments are more focused than before. There is hope for better treatments, not as harsh on your other organs. But still, the best treatment is prevention.

One very important note and the point of this book: *Cancer does not have to necessarily be killed. You can have a full life with a disease that is under control.* Same as people who do well with controlled blood pressure or controlled diabetes.

But it will not happen without trying. Educate yourself. Read, research, and act on that information. Start now.

Chapter 6

The Role of Exercise in Disease and Healing

We were born to be active, to move around, to interact with our surroundings. Plants were not. You are not a plant. So get moving.

Until the not-so-distant past, humans had to walk everywhere.

The benefits of exercise are incredible. Today, we need gyms and exercise equipment to stay active. The quarantine during the pandemic and working from home have made us more and more sedentary. Even children that we could hardly keep at home because they wanted to be outside playing, now is difficult to get them out of their bedroom, never mind to make them go to play outside.

What you eat ends up in your blood. Now blood must reach the tissues that need those nutrients. Exercise improves circulation. With improved circulation, more blood gets to the lungs, and thus, oxygen levels improve at the tissue level. As you move, the matter inside your intestines moves faster, and more stuff is emptied into your lymphatic system to be disposed of. More dopamine and serotonin, carried from your intestines to your brain, means happiness. You may find new and old friends at your exercise venue. The more positive your attitude, the better your productivity will be. The better the muscle tone, the less chance of falls. More sun, more vitamin D. It will be a whole new you!

It is important that you exercise in a way that you like and enjoy. Choose carefully here, or you will quit. I enjoy a stationary bike. Some prefer swimming. It is a very personal decision, but you must stick with it.

For those that can, a personal trainer or a more disciplined program, like Pilates or yoga, would be safer and better to stick to.

Chapter 7

Nutrition in Cancer

Emotions may contribute to cancer; detoxifying may stop growth, but it is nutrition that will kill it.

So let's talk about nutrition in general terms. Nutrients are the molecules that must enter your body to allow it to function.

I will group nutrients into four categories:

For energy
For tissue composition
For function
For cleaning (detox)

For energy. Carbohydrates (sugars) are the main source of energy for us. Glucose and fructose are the most common ones. Fructose comes from fruits and is a 5-carbon carbohydrate. Glucose is a 6-carbon molecule. Fructose cannot be converted to fat—only glucose. Sugars get inside the cell by way of insulin, testosterone, and vitamin D. The cell has an area to burn sugars for energy, the equivalent of a furnace called the *mitochondria*. A chemical reaction called the cycle of Krebs is how the body creates energy out of sugars. Thyroid function directly controls this. It should be noted that fluoride (present in city water and most toothpaste products) interferes with this function, slowing it down and creating chronic fatigue.

Cancer cells have modified their mitochondria to produce more energy. One of the treatments that I use on my patients exploits this defect and makes the cancer cell need more energy, eventually starving to death.

For tissue composition, we need calcium, vitamin C, protein, collagen, and other substances. That is why we need a variety of foods. Please rotate and have variety. A healthy salad made of the same ingredients every day is not good. There are about ninety-nine nutrients that our body needs to function. You can't eat the same things every day and expect to have all the nutrients that you need. Thus, eat different things with different nutrients so that you can have all you need for your tissues to function properly and to fight disease and heal.

For function, we need vitamins, hormones, fiber, and electrolytes. Our body produces many things out of the molecules that we eat. Some vitamins and all hormones are produced by our tissues. Not so the electrolytes. We must intake sodium, potassium, calcium, iodine, etc., constantly to stay alive.

Fiber keeps the intestinal conveyor belt moving. It also helps to trap unwanted stuff and make sure it exits the body without harming you. There are two types of fiber: soluble and insoluble. Both are essential for function.

Detoxification. The body, like an engine, produces waste while functioning. To detoxify is to remove the waste. The body will get rid of unwanted substances from the cells using glutathione, a substance that each cell produces, and antioxidants, and then dumps the waste out using the renal system (kidneys, urine), the intestinal tract (liver, feces, lymphatic system), the skin (sweat) and the lungs (breath). These systems must work at peak for your benefit. The cleaner you live, the less they have to work, and the lesser chance that you get sick. The opposite is also true: the more toxins and bad substances that enter your body, the higher the possibility of getting sick.

Drink at least sixty ounces of water a day. It is not just for hydration; it is for detox.

As you see, we are what we eat. Choose wisely.

I strongly believe in supplementation. Today's food is grown in over-harvested soil. We don't let the soil rest every seven years as mandated in the Holy Bible.

If you believe that we can get nutrients only from the food that we eat, then why is it that you don't cry anymore while cutting an onion? Peppers and tomatoes don't fill the room with smell. Today's white rice has no fiber, just carbs. These are not our grandparent's vegetables. We need supplementation. I suggest starting with a basic multivitamin and multi-mineral complex and adding individual nutrients according to your specific needs. Again, choose quality. Powered vegetables and fruits are an excellent way to supplement.

The method of cooking is also important. Cook, but don't kill your food. Extreme temperatures deactivate many chemical complexes. Pasteurization is one. The most efficient method is soup. Raw is good, but our digestive system will have a harder time extracting nutrients. Juicing is another good one. Fresh is always better. Canned foods may not be my first choice. Full of preservatives, and on top of that, metals from the can may end up in your tissues. Think of fresh and frozen foods as your first choice.

For dessert, choose fresh fruits. Yogurt will help replenish the good bacteria in your gut but is not a sufficient substitute for a prime pre/probiotic if your health is already compromised.

Only drink water that has not been treated with chlorine or fluoride, even if it says that it has been filtered and purified. I called it dead water because it can't hold memory. (We can talk about that on another occasion). I choose spring water. It is clean water filtered for particles. Distilled water is not good for you either.

If you are on well water, get it tested. Clean, safe, well water is an excellent choice.

Chapter 8

Prevention

As you may already know by reading how to fight cancer, the best thing is to prevent it, to never be diagnosed with it.

One ounce of prevention is worth a ton of cure.

What is my protocol for cancer prevention? It is simple. The earlier in life that you start implementing this plan, the better the outcome. Share this with your loved ones. Those that you don't want to see diagnosed with this disease. The best part is that it also works to prevent most acquired illnesses.

First: Be happy. You must straighten your life. Analyze, pray, talk. A certified life coach may become handy. Talk to your priest or rabbi or spiritual counselor if necessary. Whatever you have to do to have a happy, peaceful life. Get rid of a stressful job. When possible, walk away from a toxic relationship. Limit the time that you spend at work or on work-related activities. Balance is the key. Of course, we must be productive, but remember that after you die, your job will not cease. Someone will replace you. Nobody is indispensable or irreplaceable.

Time gone is time gone. Take time to enjoy the things that *you* like. It is okay to please other people, but there is nothing wrong with also pleasing yourself. Go out to eat. Buy that thing that you have been looking at for a long time. Take that trip to that special place. Go visit that friend. Spend time with your kids and grandkids. Buy that special chair and place it on the back porch to spend lazy afternoons reading and enjoying the birds and the view.

Tell your loved ones that you love them and show it: hug, kiss, share a good cup of coffee or a glass of wine or beer.

Live your life. Remember, *nobody will make it out of here alive!*

Second: Nutrition. Again, write everything you eat for three days and then do an honest evaluation. Sometimes, changes must be done gradually, like less sugar in your coffee. Get the idea in your head that you want to live healthy for a long time and change is necessary. Talk to a competent nutritionist. A naturopath physician is an excellent choice to help you. Put together a plan, then execute.

Supplement with high-quality, no-preservative, natural product. Any vitamin that the name ends in "yl" is man-made. Liquids are better absorbed than hard tablets. Powdered supplements that you mix with juice or water are highly absorbable—nothing like eating the whole fruit. You can make 100 percent natural fruit salad and eat some with each meal as your dessert.

Third: Exercise. Thirty minutes five days a week. That is all it takes to have a reasonable circulation. Be disciplined. Have an exercise plan and follow it. Remember, you don't have to spend money on this. Walking may be an excellent way to achieve an adequate level of movement. A treadmill or exercise bike are great alternatives for those days when the weather does not cooperate.

Fourth: Rest and leisure. Work is important, but it is not the reason you were born to do. Yes, be productive and be the best employee/executive/owner ever, but don't take work home. Learn to prioritize and to delegate. Take deep breaths to get more oxygen to your brain, and make wise decisions. Plan your work schedule. Plan your vacation time so you have something to look forward to. Never skip meals. It's not worth it, and in the end, it will not make any difference. Have your doctor check your testosterone levels (both males and females). This is very important for your efficiency at work. You can check our web page to learn more about Executive Brain Optimization.

Only in America, we have thirty-minute lunches. That is not enough time to look at the menu. In Spain, the lunch break is three to four hours. Yes, you read right. Long lunches. People go back home, eat, take a nap, and then go back to work and relax for another very productive four hours. The idea is to not be in a hurry. The Lord is not going to say: "Oh, poor Joe, he spent thirty minutes doing something that he didn't have to do. Let's delay the time to come back to heaven by thirty minutes." No, when your time is up, your time is up. Spend it wisely.

Fifth: Have regular checkups. Abnormalities can show during routine testing before symptoms appear. I prefer thermography to regular mammograms for early detection of breast cancer and other conditions.

Hormones should be checked on everybody after thirty-five. Our poor health habits are making our bodies fail earlier, producing imbalances at younger ages.

Men need their prostate health checked by a blood test called PSA (prostate specific antigen). This test can detect prostate gland problems five years before cancer can be felt on a rectal exam. Save yourself the embarrassment, and you may even save your life by early detection. Prostate enlargement can also affect the quality of life as it contributes to many trips to the bathroom at night.

I use quantum resonance to diagnose in a non-invasive way. It gives us a lot of information in a short time in a very inexpensive way.

Regular checkups should not be limited to cancer. EKGs check for heart conditions, blood work may show diabetes, thyroid problems, anemia, hormone imbalance, etc.

Chapter 9

Last Word

Well, here I stop, and you continue. It has been my pleasure to bring essential information to you. Now is your opportunity to turn knowledge into action.

A lot can be done to stop or control this disease. But it all starts and ends with the patient. You have cancer. Not your doctor. Not your relatives. You.

The support system is there. The information is there. Use common sense. Don't let the cure be worse than the disease.

A condition called cancer has claimed the lives of many of my patients and relatives.

Enough!

I have decided to do something about it. A copy of the book that you just read is going to all my living relatives. I don't want to lose anybody else to this totally preventable and treatable health issue.

Please seek a physician who knows how to prevent your beautiful and healthy cells from mutating into ugly cancer cells. Don't wait for a diagnosis before you are evaluated. An ounce of prevention is worth a ton of cure.

Have a good, comprehensive physical if you don't have symptoms.

And have a focused examination if something doesn't just feel right. Be one step ahead when it comes to your health.

If you are already diagnosed with cancer, after reading this book, you should know that there is a way to fight back. Whatever you do, for your sake and those who love you and depend on you, DON'T GIVE UP WITHOUT A FIGHT!

It is important that you don't fear cancer but take it head-on. Change bad habits for good ones, and review your health status at least once a year or as soon as a symptom or suspicion appears.

Don't be afraid of telling a competent surgeon: "Sir, take this damn thing out of me ASAP." Then rush to find out how and why it developed to prevent it from ever coming back again.

These suggestions do not take the place of a regular diagnosis and treatment plan with your personal doctor and oncologist. Most of my cancer patients come to me while under oncology treatment, seeking a parallel protocol. The oncologist should be aware of what you do besides his anti-cancer treatment.

Research shows that patients may do better when they take advantage of both traditional medicine and regenerative medicine than when they follow just one type of treatment.

Now is the time for you to say:

My dear cancer cells, it is time for you to go, and if you stay in me, I expect you to behave and not interfere with my happiness. I don't have any more time for you. I have decided to live my life without worries.

I pray for the Lord to give you health and wisdom. To give you strength and a support system to help you navigate these difficult times and to carry you safely to a place called health.

Visit our website, Jimmydiazmd.com, for more information and also to place yourself on our prayer list.

The best to you!

Jimmy Diaz, MD, and our
Health Restoration Team

About the Author

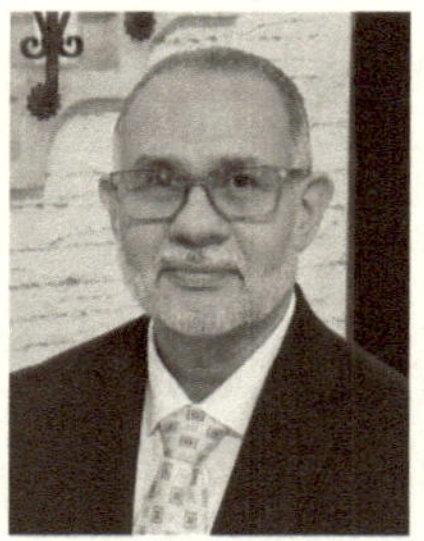

Dr. Jimmy Diaz has practiced medicine for over thirty-five years. His first specialty is in internal medicine, and in the last twenty years, he has trained and practiced functional regenerative medicine. During this period, he has treated many cancer patients in various stages of the disease. In his office in the city of Alpharetta, a suburb of Atlanta in the state of Georgia, USA, patients visit him from every state and foreign countries.

Dr. Diaz focuses on the cause of a disease, not the symptoms, and takes pride in his training in the field of alternative medicine. By joining that expertise together with the field of modern medicine, he approaches each patient as an individual, not as a client, in order to eliminate the ailment from the root, at the cellular level.

Now semiretired, he lives in the Caribbean Island of Puerto Rico. Sitting by the beach, he gets inspiration to write for patients and prepares conferences for his colleagues to pass on his vast knowledge in disease prevention and treatment with minimal intervention and minimal side effects.

His emphasis is on helping people to survive the terrible illness called cancer so that they can go on and live a happy life, even if they cannot get rid of the disease.